How to I
Sexuality a.
15 Secrets That Will Keep Her Coming
Back for More!

You've been lied to. Women LOVE sex! The problem is, what works for most men is opposite of what works for most women.

In this revolutionary Itty Bitty Book, Jan Robinson lifts the veils on feminine sexuality, and shows you how to stop wasting time with clichéd approaches that don't work and start focusing on what does so that you both get to enjoy more great sex more often.

You will learn:
- The little-known universal principles that underlie female sexual arousal.

- Practical techniques for sparking deep-level attraction and igniting her desire.

- Secrets to unlocking a woman's orgasmic response and giving her full-body orgasms, every time.

Pick up a copy of this eye-opening book and discover new paths to mind-blowing, soul-satisfying, ultimately fulfilling sex.

Your Amazing
Itty Bitty®
Have More Sex
Book

*15 Secrets to Satisfying Your Partner and
Having Her Come Back for More!*

Jan Robinson

Published by Itty Bitty® Publishing
A subsidiary of S & P Productions, Inc.

Printed in the United States of America

Itty Bitty® Publishing
311 Main Street, Suite E
El Segundo, CA 90245
(310) 640-8885

ISBN: 978-1-931191-74-6

This book is dedicated to all of my dear teachers and mentors, students and clients, lovers and beloveds, all who have guided me closer to an understanding of the nature of love, Divine consciousness, and the mysteries of sexuality.

Stop by our Itty Bitty® website to find interesting blog entries regarding better sex and intimacy.

www.IttyBittyPublishing.com

Or visit Jan Robinson at
www.magicsex.us

Want to learn more? You're invited to this no-cost virtual seminar: "3 Massive Mistakes Most Men Make That KILL a Woman's Desire for Sex" (And What To Do Instead!).

Access this FREE online presentation at:

www.havemoresexbook/
3massivemistakes

Table of Contents

Introduction

In this Itty Bitty. Book you will find 15 secrets
for having and enjoying better, hotter, and more
frequent sex.

Secrets 1 and 2 lay out the radical keys to
unleashing any woman's naturally wild sexual
side. Secrets 3-6 give you fool-proof tips and
techniques for creating connection and sparking
deep attraction. Secrets 7-11 answer the question
of how to get her in the mood and ramp up her
desire through electrifying foreplay and
seduction. Secrets 12-15 focus on intercourse and
how to make sex sizzle.

So, the question is, why DON'T women keep
coming back for more? I mean, what's there not
to like, right? I'm about to tell you something that
is going to change your sex life, forever.

You've been lied to.

Women LOVE sex! In fact, the masculine energy
within you has the power to awaken the luscious
sexuality that lives inside of her.

Every woman has a sex kitten inside of her. She
may be hiding out and too uncomfortable or
afraid to come out of her cage, but, I assure you,
these step-by-step approaches will have her
feeling safe and ready to express her carnal
desires with you.

This book will give you new insights into feminine sexuality and help you support the special woman in your life as she awakens to the glory of her sexual power.

In the process, you'll become better, a more powerful and sensitive lover, as you discover that, once you tap into a woman's capacity for infinite pleasure, you will find yourself on an ascending virtuous circle of relating. Her turn-on will fuel your turn-on, which will in turn fuel hers, and then yours, and so on, propelling you to ever new heights together.

You will be amazed.

Discover how implementing even a little from the following secrets goes a long way. Enjoy!

Secret 1
The Surprising Keys to Unlock Her Lust

When it comes to getting a woman to want to have sex with you again and again (and again), the most dangerous mistake is "doing what comes naturally." What works for most women is opposite of what works for most men. Here are some of the unexpected keys that reliably unlock her lust.

1. Heart to Sex. A woman becomes most available sexually once she's fulfilled emotionally. Romance works!
2. Responsive vs. Spontaneous. For a woman, desire for sex doesn't typically appear "out of the blue." Her arousal depends upon a context that stimulates it.
3. Sensual vs. Visual. Her sexuality is aroused through her sensual and emotional channels more so than her visual and mental ones.
4. Like Water, Not Fire. Unlike a man's fiery sexual response, a woman's sexual nature is like water: slow to reach the boiling point, but long to hold the heat.
5. Process vs. Goal Oriented. More important to a woman's sexual fulfillment is not the sequence of the activities, the WHAT, but the quality of those activities, that is, the HOW.

The Paradox of Feminine Sexuality

- Remember this: The initial stimulus leading to a woman's sexual turn-on is generally *not* sexual in nature.
- Most men will never be aware of or understand this paradox and therefore remain forever in the dark about the truth of where his wife's or girlfriend's sexual desire actually comes from.
- Have you ever asked your partner, "Honey, tell me what you want, tell me what excites you" and not gotten very far? This is normal. She probably doesn't know herself!!
- The point is, a woman's sexual response does not operate in a direct and overt way, like a man's.
- What turns a man on sexually is generally sexual in nature (*e.g.* you see a woman naked—it turns you on, she reaches for your cock—it turns you on).
- For a woman, there is almost always an intermediary between the arousing stimulus and her sexual turn-on.
- That intermediary is her HEART. (*e.g.* you massage her feet—it touches her heart—it turns her on; you bring her a red rose—it touches her heart—it turns her on).
- Energy passes first from her heart center and then to her sex center.

Secret 2
Her 5 Sexual Desire Triggers

There are 5 things most women must have in order to open and abandon herself sexually to you. Women *deeply* long to feel:

1. Emotionally Close and Connected—Care for her through your time, attention, and gestures of non-sexual affection.
2. Safe and Relaxed—Be emotionally available, honest, trustworthy, and authentic. Your integrity and presence are what has her feel secure in the relationship.
3. Appreciated and Special—Shower her with compliments. Make her feel special by expressing your love to her via her primary love language[1].
4. Feminine and Sexy—Pay attention to and praise what you find beautiful, womanly, and irresistible about her!
5. Ecstatically Awakened and Liberated— Bring her to levels of pleasure she didn't know herself capable of through slow seduction and prolonged lovemaking.

♂

---

[1] Chapman, Gary D. The Five Love Languages: How to Express Heartfelt Commitment to Your Mate. Northfield Publishing, 2004.

The Non-Linear Model of the Female Sexual Response

- In 1966 Masters and Johnson came out with their theory of a four-stage model for the human sexual response: arousal, plateau, orgasm and resolution.
- The problem is, it assumed that male and female sexual responses both operate in a similar, linear fashion.
- In 1997, prominent female sex researchers[2] presented a circular model that acknowledged the key role that pleasure and satisfaction play in a woman's desire. If sex resulted in pleasure and satisfaction, another encounter would likely follow. But if it didn't, it would likely lead to fewer ones.
- In 2001, a non-linear model was published that acknowledged non-sexual factors such as emotional intimacy, sensual stimuli, and relationship satisfaction as essential to a woman's turn-on.
- In short, the female sex drive is largely *responsive* rather than spontaneous. That means, women typically won't make the first move, because they actually *need* your advances in order to get turned on.

---

[2] Judy Norsigian et al. Our Bodies Our Selves: A New Edition for a New Era. Simon and Schuster, 2005.

Secret 3
The #1 Secret to Avoid or Escape the Friend Zone/Roommate Syndrome

Developing your masculine presence is the single most important thing you can do to increase women's sexual desire for you. This is easy to overlook because most men are overly focused on what to do rather than how to be. Masculine presence is a practice and a way of being that you can cultivate.

1. Take up a martial art or other physical discipline that gives you primal satisfaction and builds your self-confidence.
2. Make meditation a regular part of your life to cultivate inner calm, higher awareness and mastery over your mind.
3. Learn how to hold proper eye contact with women. It will help you gain confidence and generate sexual tension.
4. Join a men's group, or lead one, and spend time with other men you admire and respect.
5. Discover your life purpose and live it fully, no excuses.
6. Cut down on addictive porn watching and learn to circulate your sexual energy. Doing so will make you a total woman magnet!

The 4 Archetypes of the Mature Masculine[3]

Seek to embody the attitudes and attributes of each archetype to become the man you want to be. Women *long* to give herself to a man whom she trusts and respects, in other words, a man who embodies the archetypes in their fullness.

- **The Lover***:* sensual, passionate, adventurous, emotionally aware, full of life.
- **The Magician:** intellectually curious, discerning, master of technologies, spiritual.
- **The Warrior**: skillful, adaptable, decisive, disciplined, takes swift and forceful initiative.
- **The King**: centered, protective, deliberate, principled, in integrity, blesses and empowers others.
- **The Lover** *(underdeveloped):* womanizing, obsessed, depressed, misogynistic, workaholic.
- **The Magician** *(underdeveloped):* manipulative, lazy, begrudging, cynical.
- **The Warrior** *(underdeveloped):* emotionally numb, martyr, passive aggressive, abusive.
- **The King** *(underdeveloped)*: irresponsible, bullying, controlling, cruel, narcissistic.

---

[3] Moore, Douglas. Rediscovering the Archetypes of the Mature Masculine. Harper Collins, 1990.

Secret 4
The Foundation of Attraction

What can you do to generate a sense of connection and magic spark with a woman, whether you're on a first date or waking up to your wife of twelve years? Knowing how to establish rapport is the foundational step for building and sustaining attraction and desire.

1. Use the match and mirror techniques for building rapport. This will have a woman feel close and comfortable with you.
2. Mirror her body language. Start with the overall posture and placement of the limbs, then smaller gesticulations, and lastly the more subtle expressions of her eyes and face.
3. Echo her words. To let her know you "get" her, repeat the main point of the last thing she said using her wording.
4. Match the tempo, resonance and volume of her voice. More important than the words you say is HOW you say them.
5. To deepen the intimacy of conversation, ask her plenty of open-ended questions (*i.e.* "What was the best thing about your day today?" "What are you passionate about in your life right now?").

Breaking Rapport to Intensify Attraction

- Don't be boring. Too much comfort and familiarity will undermine attraction and land you in the friend zone, or worse, in a sexless marriage.
- "Nice guys" tend to be good at building rapport, but bad at breaking it, which is essential for sparking attraction ("Jerks," do the opposite).
- You don't have to be a jerk in order for a woman to want you. It's about being creative and confident enough in yourself to take interpersonal risks.
- Once you have a warm connection, break rapport on occasion, unexpectedly change up the dynamic in playful ways.
- Body language: If you've been sitting and leaning in towards her during conversation, lean back.
- Conversational Leadership. If the mood is flat, stir things up. Raise or lower the volume of your speaking, tell a funny story, or start a new conversational thread with a strong opinion.
- Boundaries. A woman will respect you when you communicate your honest needs and desires in a calm, clear way (*e.g.* "You know what? I really don't want to talk about this topic. Let's talk about something else.").
- Dare to be bold. Acts of boldness spike dopamine which fuels attraction.

Secret 5
The Power of Body Language

Being aware of your own body language gives you the advantage to increase attraction and convey confidence. Here are eight simple nonverbal cues that bypass a woman's critical mind and stimulate her limbic system, the part of the brain that regulates sexual arousal

1. Smile. Smiling shows a woman that you're confident, friendly, approachable.
2. Move and walk deliberately. Don't make unnecessary, jerky or fidgety movements.
3. Maintain an open posture. Uncross your arms, keep an open stance with your legs.
4. Stand tall and straight, keeping your shoulders back, your chest open.
5. Lift your chin slightly, bring your head back and keep your eyes forward and open.
6. Make eye contact and don't be the first one to look away. Don't dart your eyes around when speaking with her.
7. Start with brief touches (elbow, knee, shoulder, back); move to flirtatious touch (hugging, stroking); and then to more intimate gestures (hair, face, neck).
8. Appeal to women's keen sense of smell. You want your hair, face, and body scent to work for you, not against you.

How Do I Know If She's In the Mood?

As a guy who's either single or married, you're continually having to deal with the possibility of rejection. Increase your chances and avoid missing out on opportunities by knowing the subtle body language cues that signal she's interested in you and in the mood.

- When you're in conversation, her feet are pointing toward you, not angled away.
- She gestures in ways that release her pheromones: tossing and playing with her hair, tilting the head, exposing her neck, touching her neck or upper chest.
- She visibly or audibly responds when you touch her: she sighs, wiggles, moves in closer to you, touches you back.
- She smiles and looks happy. She looks at you. Her breathing is relaxed and open.
- She creates opportunities for physical closeness, suggests spending time together, asks for cuddles or a shoulder or foot rub.
- If she's not demonstrating any of these attraction cues, assess and recalibrate. Too much comfort and not enough spark? Coming on too strong and not enough rapport?

Secret 6
A Man's Kiss Is His Signature

There's one thing that, above all else, will instantly turn a woman either on or off: Your kiss. Knowing the secrets to lip-locking magic is a sure-fire way to prime her passion for more.

1. Relax the muscles of your lips, tongue, face, and jaw.
2. Push your lips forward slightly to make them soft and pillowy.
3. Stay shallow and light at first. Softly brush your lips over hers to build anticipation and excitement.
4. Open your mouth slightly, keeping your lips just barely parted.
5. Breathe as you kiss.
6. Keep it slow and sensual. Act like you have all the time in the world. The kiss will speed up and intensify on its own.
7. Mix things up by alternating speed, pressure, depth and the modality of kiss.
8. Creatively use all 5 kissing modalities: lipping, tonguing, blowing, sucking, biting.
9. Put your body and emotions behind your kiss. Use your hands, hold her, stroke her face and body, subtlely move your pelvis forward and back to turn up the heat.

The 12 Worst Kissing Mistakes

One of the first marriage warning signs is when the kissing stops. And if you're single and dating, 65-80% of women won't give a bad kisser a second date. Avoid the following:

- Tight lips and stiff tongue.
- Aggressively going in for fully open-mouthed kiss right off the bat.
- Missing your target: not meeting the pillowy parts of her lips with yours.
- Pressing too hard with your lips.
- Going too fast.
- Same old same old.
- Getting slobbery: too much tongue action without any lip movement.
- Sucking too hard on her tongue.
- Not using your hands for holding, cradling, caressing, stroking her face and body.
- Forgetting to breathe.
- Bad breath.
- Approaching kissing as a perfunctory means to an end rather than as a luscious and satisfying experience unto itself. Rediscover the magic and power of kissing and give her a preview of what's to come!

Secret 7
Foreplay: "What's In It for ME?"

If the woman in your life is far less interested in sex than you are, it means that, for her, the sex she's having isn't sex worth wanting. The right kind of foreplay reliably awakens her desire and lust. The better the foreplay, the hotter and more memorable the sex.

1. Great foreplay has three components, in this specific order: 1) emotional intimacy, 2) full-body sensuality, and 3) stimulation of her primary sex points.
2. Don't go straight for her tits and clit. *Ever.* It will short-circuit her sexual energy, short-change her pleasure, and ultimately limit her ability to orgasm. Tease her instead.
3. Good foreplay IS seduction. The purpose of seduction is to open a woman sexually, just like the warmth of the sun inspires a flower blossom to open.
4. Women need a *minimum* of 20 minutes to become fully aroused. It needn't happen every time, just more often than not.
5. Base your foreplay/seduction approach on one of her erotic blueprints (Secret 12) leading her to the deepest arousal, most intense sexual desire, and full-body orgasm.

The "Quickie" Foreplay Formula

- This potent seduction formula is based upon natural energy flows. First, they relax a woman's body - a necessary precursor for her sexual turn-on. Then they stimulate her.
- To Relax Her: Have your partner lie face down on a bed, floor pad, or massage table. Sweep your hands down all the back and side surfaces of her body, from above her head to out the tips of her fingers and toes.
- To Stimulate Her: Have her roll onto her back and do a three-part sensual massage up the front surface of her body, from the soles of her feet to out through her fingertips or the top of her head.
- Part One: sensually stroke up her body, from feet to head, bypassing her primary erogenous zones (genitals, breasts, nipples, lips) which will heighten her anticipation.
- Part Two: From her feet out through the tips of her fingers, kiss and caress her body; include the periphery of her primary sex points, but without direct stimulation.
- Part Three: From feet to head, stimulate her body, include her sex points this time, but then move on from those areas to leave her aching for more…

Secret 8
Hacking Her Inner Love Pharmacy

Studies show that sex begins and ends in the brain. The most important neurotransmitter you need to know about is the "love drug," oxytocin. Help your partner's brain produce more oxytocin and she will be far more responsive to you sexually.

1. When a woman is feeling safe, relaxed, and in love, copious amounts of oxytocin are flowing from her brain and she feels most available for sexual connection.
2. When a woman is feeling unsafe (physically or emotionally) and stressed out, oxytocin production stops and cortisol (the stress hormone) kicks in.
3. Cortisol produces a protein that binds to all the available testosterone in her bloodstream which KILLS her sex drive.
4. This is why, when a woman is dealing with job pressure, family problems, or a relationship issue, sex is the LAST thing on her mind.
5. For men, sex occurs as a fine solution to a stressful day! For women, it doesn't. Oxytocin production is the key to turn things around. And THEN the option for sex is back on the table. Woo hoo!

10 Ways to Give Any Woman the Big "O"!

- Give her random hugs, physical affection, kissing at times when you are not wanting sex.
- Buy her chocolate or bring her flowers for no reason.
- Take her out shopping for a new outfit, new pair of shoes or lingerie.
- Meditate, breathe and cuddle together.
- Take a walk together holding hands.
- Laugh together often (women prefer men who make them laugh).
- Put on her favorite music and dance her around the room.
- Enjoy activities with friends (i.e. wine tasting, hosting a dinner party, going out dancing, hiking in nature).
- Ask her how her day went and really listen. Put your full attention on her, sit with her and touch her affectionately. Be patient and genuinely curious. Deepen the conversation with questions like, "How did that make you feel?" "What was that like?" "What else would you like to share?... anything else?"
- Clean house (a.k.a. "female porn." New research proves that men who share equal housework enjoy more sex with their wives).

Secret 9
Prime Her Emotions for Explosive Sex

Women need to feel emotional safety and trust with their partner in order to allow themselves full sexual abandon. That means, the more skillfully you know how to navigate difficult emotions with your mate when they arise, the more passionately she'll open up to you when it comes time for sex.

1. Be proactive: as soon as you notice she's upset, approach her in a caring manner and initiate a conversation. You can say, "You seem upset, hon. Tell me what's going on."
2. When a woman is emotional, she needs to feel listened to by you, understood, and nurtured by your loving attention.
3. Focus on these three things: 1) non-judgmental listening, 2) giving her the space to express what she's thinking and feeling without interruption, and 3) letting her know you understand what she's saying and feeling.
4. Simple forms of physical affection like holding her hand work wonders.
5. Use phrases such as "Take as much time as you need. I'm here for you." "How can I support you right now?"

Pitfalls and Phrases to Avoid

TIP: Resisting her emotions, ignoring or avoiding her until she's no longer upset, minimizing her problems, offering unsolicited advice or solutions, invalidating or trying to talk her out of her feelings, or getting upset that she's upset only add fuel to the fire. Avoid the following phrases:

- "You're blowing things out of proportion."
- "You're overreacting."
- "You're making a big deal out of nothing."
- "This is too much."
- "Why are you getting so upset about this?" ("Why" questions will put her on the defensive).
- "It's no big deal."
- "It's really not all that bad."
- "Please don't cry."
- "Pull yourself together."
- "You're too sensitive."
- "Are you getting your period?"
- "Can we drop this now?"
- "I can't win with you!"
- "What do you want me to say?!"
- "Can we have make-up sex now?" (Avoid asking for sex. It's generally a turn-off. Instead, once she's feeling close and relaxed with you again, invite her *non-verbally* through sensual, passionate seduction).

Secret 10
The Power of Touch

Of the things a woman really needs in order to desire sex with you again and again, touch is the ONLY means that can fulfill all of them. Here are her five sexual desire triggers and tips for how you can satisfy them through your touch.

1. Emotionally Close and Connected: Hold hands, caress her cheek with the back of your hand, make warming circles on the back of her heart (clockwise motion).
2. Safe and Relaxed: Hold her on your lap and stroke her hair, give her a shoulder rub, spoon with her and breathe with her in sync.
3. Appreciated and Special: Kiss her forehead, take the time to caress her non-sexual parts. This will have her feeling appreciated for ALL of her.
4. Feminine and Sexy: Caress feather-light over all her curves, rub, press and tap on her sacrum bone, cup her breasts and vulva with slow or non-moving touch.
5. Sexually Awakened and Liberated. Do the "Quickie Foreplay Formula" (Secret 7) followed by a 45-90 minute "Pussy massage" (Secret 11).

Guidelines for Electrifying Touch

Want to spoil her for other men and "divorce-proof" your relationship? Touch her body better than anyone else. Develop your quality of touch by following these guidelines:

- Breathe fully and freely as you touch, in through the nose and out through the mouth. The more you breathe, the more pleasure she feels.
- SLOW DOWN enough to feel pleasurable sensation in your own hands as you touch. In other words, don't worry about making her happy; make your hands happy. It'll ensure a touch that feels very connected.
- Bring emotion into your touch. Convey love, nurturing, tenderness, desire, passion through your hands. Visualize or imagine "glowing" the warmth of your love into your partner's body.
- Alternate speed and pressure (slow, fast, soft and firm stimulation) to create variety and trigger her brain to release feel-good endorphins.
- Avoid monotony. Don't use only one type of stroke over and over. Vary the modalities of your touch: sometimes caress, then squeeze and press, gently tap or lightly scratch, vibrate, rock and roll. Keep her mind guessing and you'll raise her anticipation to a fever pitch!

Secret 11
The BEST Way to Make a Woman Sexually Happy

As a man, you have the sacred privilege to help awaken a woman to the infinite erotic and sexual potential that lies within her. A woman has NO IDEA of the ecstatic pleasure her body is capable of until she meets a man who can liberate her orgasmic response through a long, slow, attentive pussy (or "yoni") massage.

1. Bathe her and bring her into a heated room with soft candle light and music.
2. Give her a slow, sensual body massage.
3. Rest your hands on her heart center and vulva. Tell her know how pretty her pussy is (really!) Look into her eyes.
4. Take your time exploring external strokes. LESS IS MORE.
5. Before you move to internal massage strokes, ask her permission, "May I enter you?" (Those are healing words).
6. Invite her to tell you when she feels spots that are numb, burning or pinched. Hold those while breathing fully until you feel a pulsation arise and pleasurable, healing sensations flow in.
7. Alternate healing strokes with pleasurable ones (include her clitoris).
8. Exit slowly and spoon with her.

4 Essential Pussy Massage Strokes

- Heart-Vulva Connect. Cup her vulva in one hand while resting your other hand over her heart, on the sternum bone, between her nipples. Relax your fingers, look into her eyes, breathe.
- The Pussy Pet. Using a hand-over-hand technique and a generous amount of massage oil, stroke from her vaginal opening up over her clitoris. Experiment with various levels of speed and pressure.
- The Crescent. Glide your ring finger into her vagina, palm facing up. Rotate your wrist side to side so that you are describing a crescent shape with the pad of your finger. Stimulate the upper, lower, and side walls of her vagina.
- Finding the G-Spot. Once she is very aroused, enter her vagina with your middle finger, palm facing upward. Applying medium pressure with the pad of your finger make repeated "come hither" gestures deliberately from back to front, left to right over the G-Spot Area. This area is a small section of erectile tissue on the upper wall of the vagina. The ribbed texture here differs from the surrounding tissue which is smooth and velvety. You have found the G-Spot itself when her eyes practically bug out from the intense sensation. Give this sensitive area prolonged focused stimulation.

Secret 12
Navigating Her Erotic Blueprints

Knowing the paths to her turn-ons better than she knows herself is a sure-fire way to give her more pleasure than she's ever known before. Similar to the underwater currents that exist in the ocean, there are natural energy flows in a woman's subtle body. You can't see them, but they are there. Here are three primary blueprints:

1. Periphery to Center. To best arouse and seduce a woman, focus the stimulation at the periphery of her body first (head, hands, and feet) and then systematically work your way to her center (nipples and genitals).
2. Down the Back and Up the Front. Brush down the back surface of the body to relax her and stroke sensually up the front of the body to stimulate and excite her. Bypass her primary sex points in the first pass, then gradually include them in your second and third (See Secret 7).
3. Sexual Reflexology Zones. Relax her body and raise her libido by giving her a foot rub and tracing over the highly erogenous areas of her feet: around the ankle bones, across the ankle crease, sides of the heels, and on the big toe.

When to Enter Her?

The Taoists, who have one of the world's great ancient wisdom traditions around sex, have a couple of clever sayings when it comes to the question of when it's time to move to penetration sex.

- "Don't float your boat in a rocky river." And "Don't throw your peas in before your carrots."
- That means, don't penetrate her until her sexual juices are flowing. And, take the time to warm her up through unrushed foreplay because you (peas) heat up faster than she does (carrots).
- Ready, set, SLOW! Making her wait for penetration creates some of the most exciting moments for her during sex.
- Three signs that she's ready: 1) "Puffy" outer lips (the "vestibular bulbs"); 2) Increase in pitch and volume of her sounds; 3) Bowing and arching of her back, or pulling you closer in to her by grabbing your butt cheeks or wrapping her legs around you.

Secret 13
The Ultimate Secret to Mind-Blowing Orgasms: Hers and Yours!

Developing the skills to hold your ejaculation and last longer is the number one most important technique you'll ever learn to improve your sexual performance and satisfy your partner. If you can't last more than 20 minutes, your partner won't experience her full potential for vaginal, multiple and ejaculatory ("squirting") orgasms.

1. The average man lasts only 4-7 minutes during penetration sex. Most women need 15-45 minutes to reach orgasm.
2. Most women don't know what they're missing out on when all they've known is quick sex. Be the exception for her.
3. A sexually awakened woman will never tell you she's disappointed that you've finished before she's even gotten started.
4. Having powerful sexual stamina gives you confidence and increases your performance.
5. If she is wanting you to finish quickly, it's a bad sign. Be sure you're taking the time to activate her five sexual desire triggers (Secret 2). Give her regular pussy massages so she can learn to enjoy the magic of prolonged lovemaking with you (Secret 11)

❀

4 Easy Steps to Delay Ejaculation

- When you feel you are approaching the brink of orgasm, the "point of no return," pause the stimulation.
- Take a long and gentle breath in through your nose and firmly press the mid-point between the anus and the scrotum, using the three longest fingers of your dominant hand.
- Angle your fingers up and back so that you are aiming the pressure toward the prostate gland.
- Hold the pressure for about 20-30 seconds while breathing gently in and out through the nose.
- Once you feel the urgency to ejaculate has diminished, release the hold and continue the stimulation.
- This simple manual technique is a great one to start out with. In order to achieve stamina for UNLIMITED sex, however, and the power to ride wave after wave of her orgasms requires mastery of the more potent internal delay techniques. Fortunately, these are techniques and skills every man can learn!

Discover more at:
www.ultimatesexualstamina.com/
lastlongertonight

Secret 14
How to Double the Chances of Giving Her a Penetration Orgasm

Varying the depth, rate, angle, and rhythm of penetration is the most easy and thrilling way to spice things up and instantly enhance your partner's erotic pleasure, while also helping you to last longer. Consider not only how your strokes feel to your penis, but also to your partner.

1. Create a magic moment by entering her slowly while looking into her eyes.
2. Start with slow, shallow strokes to heighten her anticipation and maximize her lubrication. The majority of nerve endings in the vagina are concentrated in the first two inches.
3. Move to deep strokes once she's more relaxed and aroused.
4. Alternate shallow thrusts with a single deep stroke to take her breath away.
5. Thrust at different angles in the same position in order to stimulate different parts of the vagina. Try riding high and low, angling left and right.
6. Eventually, establishing a steady pace with even rhythm for an extended period is the key to bringing her to orgasm.
7. Exit her slowly, with gratitude and awareness.

Ancient Taoist Thrusting Sequence

- Follow this classic thrusting pattern to send her over the edge. Take your time with this (faster isn't better) and breathe in a relaxed manner throughout.

  9 shallow -- 1 deep
  8 shallow -- 2 deep
  7 shallow -- 3 deep
  6 shallow -- 4 deep
  5 shallow -- 5 deep
  4 shallow -- 6 deep
  3 shallow -- 7 deep
  2 shallow -- 8 deep
  1 shallow -- 9 deep

- If you're able to perform all nine steps of the sequence, continue in the reverse order.

Secret 15
"Look Into My Eyes:" Orgasmic Hypnosis to Keep Her Coming Back for More

As a woman approaches and experiences orgasm, her mind enters into a heightened state of receptivity and suggestibility. Speaking words of love and empowerment to her during the peak of her pleasure penetrates her psyche deeply, will drive her over the edge with excitement, and make sex even more amazing for the both of you.

1. Thank her. Let her know how *loved* you feel by her having opened to you sexually. Hearing this will delight her and boost her confidence.
2. Connect with her emotionally through your words. As you're f*cking her deeply you can say, "Thank you for how you love me, babe" or "I'm the luckiest man in the world right now."
3. Other phrases: "You are SO beautiful in this moment, baby." "I LOVE how powerful you are!" "I love you so much!"
4. Choose your words thoughtfully, from your heart, never out of the desire to manipulate. Keep it simple and genuine.
5. Shine your love out your eyes and look deeply into hers.

The Power of Pillow Talk

Caution! Post sex, the hormone prolactin gets released which makes you want to sleep. To cement your lover's memory of a positive sexual experience and reinforce her desire to have sex with you again, don't short-change yourselves of the magic of the afterglow phase.

- Resist the temptation to automatically close your eyes and drift off to sleep, to suddenly get up and eat, turn on the TV, or reach for your phone to start texting.
- Otherwise, you risk her feeling abandoned, unloved, even used or sleazy following sex with you (an all-too common experience for women).
- Instead, re-establish with her the experience of emotional connection and intimacy.
- Let her know you relish your connection and are in no hurry, "I could just lie here with you forever."
- Share with her highlight moments, "I loved it when…"
- Smile as you look into her eyes, stroke her hair, kiss her face tenderly.
- This will deepen her relationship satisfaction. She'll look forward to the next time knowing how much sex with you not only blows her mind with incredible pleasure but opens her heart and brings the two of you closer together.

You've finished. Before you go…

Tweet/share that you finished this book.
Please star rate this book.
Reviews are solid gold to writers. Please take a few minutes to give us some itty bitty feedback on this book.

ABOUT THE AUTHOR

Jan Robinson, M.A., tantra expert and high-performance sex coach, adores foot rubs, classical music, and men who love women.

Jan is an international teacher of Tantric Kriya Yoga, inspiring lovers to activate their *kundalini*, the most powerful energy of creation. Her passion is to initiate her clients in the joys and mysteries of sexuality, merged with their hearts and minds, for ultimate sexual fulfillment.

Her mission is to end the WAR of the sexes and encourage the WOW in the dance between the masculine and feminine. Her vision is a world in which men and women know how to rock each other's worlds!

Jan is the founder of MagicSex.Us, where she reveals ancient tantric secrets for becoming a master lover and tapping into women's infinite capacity for pleasure. Mastering Jan's proven methods will spark a sex life beyond both of your wildest dreams.

If you enjoyed this Itty Bitty® book, you might also enjoy…

- **Your Amazing Itty Bitty® Self-Esteem Book** – Jade Elizabeth
- **Your Amazing Itty Bitty® Stay Young At Any Age** – Dianna Whitley
- **Your Amazing Itty Bitty® Heal Your Body Book** – Patricia Garza Pinto

And many of our other Itty Bitty® books available on line.